FLEXITARIAN

DIET

COOKBOOK

Primarily plant-based but occasionally includes meat or other animal products in moderation.

BY

MELISSA W. LUKE

INTRODUCTION

Defining Flexitarianism

Flexitarianism represents a dynamic approach to eating that prioritizes plant-based foods while allowing for occasional inclusion of meat or other animal products in moderation. At its core, flexitarianism embraces flexibility, recognizing that dietary choices can vary based on individual preferences, cultural influences, and health considerations.

Unlike strict vegetarian or vegan diets, which eschew all animal products, flexitarianism offers a middle ground, promoting a predominantly plant-centric eating pattern while permitting flexibility to incorporate small amounts of meat or fish as desired. This flexibility is not only practical but also sustainable, making it more accessible to individuals who may be hesitant to adopt strict dietary restrictions.

The essence of flexitarianism lies in its emphasis on plant-based foods, including fruits, vegetables, whole grains, legumes, nuts, and seeds. These nutrient-dense foods form the foundation of the diet, providing essential vitamins, minerals, fiber, and antioxidants. By prioritizing plant foods, flexitarians naturally increase their intake of beneficial nutrients while reducing their reliance on heavily processed and animal-based foods.

However, what sets flexitarianism apart is its acknowledgment of the role of animal products in the diet. While some adherents may choose to eliminate meat entirely, others may opt to include occasional servings of poultry, fish, eggs, or dairy products. The key is moderation and mindfulness, focusing on the quality, sourcing, and portion size of animal products consumed.

Flexitarianism is not just about what you eat but also about how you approach food and nutrition. It encourages mindful eating, listening to your body's hunger and fullness cues, and savoring the flavors and textures of your meals. It also promotes sustainability and environmental awareness, recognizing the impact of food choices on the planet and supporting practices that minimize harm to the environment and promote animal welfare.

Ultimately, flexitarianism offers a balanced and adaptable approach to eating that can be tailored to individual needs and preferences. Whether you're looking to improve your health, reduce your environmental footprint, or simply explore new culinary horizons, embracing a flexitarian lifestyle can empower you to make positive changes while enjoying a diverse and satisfying diet.

The Benefits of a Flexitarian Approach

Improved Health: Flexitarianism has been associated with numerous health benefits. By focusing primarily on plant-based foods, flexitarians tend to consume higher levels of fiber, vitamins, and minerals, which are essential for overall health and well-being. Research suggests that a diet rich in fruits, vegetables, whole grains, and legumes may lower the risk of chronic diseases such as heart disease, diabetes, and certain cancers.

Weight Management: Flexitarianism can support weight management goals due to its emphasis on nutrient-dense, low-calorie foods. Plant-based meals are often lower in calories and saturated fats compared to animal-based dishes, making it easier to maintain a healthy weight. Additionally, the high fiber content of plant foods promotes satiety, reducing the likelihood of overeating.

Enhanced Digestive Health: The fiber found in plant-based foods is beneficial for digestive health, promoting regularity and preventing constipation. A diet rich in fruits, vegetables, and whole grains supports a healthy gut microbiome, which is essential for optimal digestion and immune function.

Environmental Sustainability:

Flexitarianism aligns with principles of sustainability by reducing the environmental impact of food production. Plant-based foods typically require fewer resources, such as water and land, and produce fewer greenhouse gas emissions compared to animal agriculture. By consuming more plant foods and fewer animal products, flexitarians can contribute to environmental conservation and mitigate climate change.

Ethical Considerations: Many individuals are drawn to flexitarianism for ethical reasons, such as concerns about animal welfare and the treatment of livestock. By reducing their consumption of meat and other animal products, flexitarians can support more humane and sustainable farming practices, such as pasture-raised meat or organic dairy production.

Versatility and Variety: One of the key advantages of flexitarianism is its flexibility and adaptability. Unlike strict vegetarian or vegan diets, which may limit food choices and culinary experiences, flexitarianism allows individuals to enjoy a wide variety of foods from different food groups. This versatility makes it easier to adhere to the diet long-term and promotes culinary creativity in meal planning and preparation.

Social and Cultural Acceptance: Flexitarianism offers a middle ground between vegetarianism/veganism and omnivorous diets, making it more socially acceptable and easier to adopt in various cultural and social contexts. Whether dining out with friends or attending family gatherings, flexitarians can navigate different food environments while still adhering to their dietary preferences and values.

Overall, the flexitarian approach offers a balanced and sustainable way of eating that promotes health, environmental stewardship, and ethical considerations, making it an appealing choice for individuals seeking to optimize their well-being while minimizing their impact on the planet.

Myth-busting: Dispelling Common Misconceptions

As with any dietary approach, flexitarianism is often subject to misconceptions and myths. Here, we address some common misunderstandings and provide clarity on what it truly means to follow a flexitarian lifestyle:

Myth: Flexitarians don't get enough protein.

Reality: Contrary to popular belief, plant-based diets can provide all the essential amino acids necessary for protein synthesis. Flexitarians have a variety of protein-rich options such as legumes, tofu, tempeh, nuts, seeds, and whole grains. Additionally, incorporating small amounts of animal products occasionally can supplement protein intake if desired.

Myth: Flexitarianism is only for vegetarians who occasionally eat meat.

Reality: While flexitarianism does involve reducing meat consumption, it is not exclusive to former vegetarians. Flexitarianism is a flexible approach to eating that can be adopted by individuals at any stage of their dietary journey, whether they currently consume meat regularly or not.

Myth: Flexitarian diets are boring and restrictive.

Reality: Flexitarianism encourages diversity and creativity in food choices. With a wide array of plant-based ingredients and culinary techniques available, flexitarians have endless possibilities for flavorful and satisfying meals. Flexitarianism is about abundance, not deprivation.

Myth: Flexitarianism is not effective for weight loss.

Reality: Flexitarianism can support weight loss and weight management goals by promoting a diet rich in nutrient-dense, low-calorie foods. By focusing on plant-based meals and moderating intake of animal products, flexitarians can create a calorie deficit while still feeling satisfied and nourished.

Myth: Flexitarians must give up their favorite meat-based dishes.

Reality: Flexitarianism is not about deprivation or giving up foods you love. Instead, it's about making conscious choices to prioritize plant-based foods while occasionally indulging in meat or other animal products in moderation. Many traditional meat-based dishes can be adapted to include more plant-based ingredients without sacrificing flavor or satisfaction.

Myth: Flexitarianism is unsustainable in the long term.

Reality: Flexitarianism is highly sustainable both for individuals and the planet. Its flexible nature allows for gradual dietary changes and adjustments over time, making it easier to maintain in the long term. Additionally, by reducing meat consumption and supporting sustainable farming practices, flexitarians contribute to environmental conservation efforts.

By dispelling these common misconceptions, we hope to provide a clearer understanding of what it means to embrace a flexitarian lifestyle. Whether you're motivated by health, environmental, or ethical considerations, flexitarianism offers a practical and sustainable approach to eating that can benefit both individuals and the planet.

Table of Contents

CHAPTER 1
GETTING STARTED: TRANSITIONING TO A FLEXITARIAN DIET

Assessing Your Current Eating Habits

Before embarking on any dietary changes, it's essential to take a close look at your current eating habits. This self-assessment can provide valuable insights into your dietary patterns, preferences, and areas for improvement. Here are some key steps to help you assess your current eating habits:

Keep a Food Journal: Start by keeping track of everything you eat and drink for several days or a week. Be sure to include all meals, snacks, and beverages, along with portion sizes and any condiments or extras. A food journal can help you become more aware of your eating patterns and identify any recurring trends or habits.

Review Nutritional Intake: Once you have a record of your food choices, review your nutritional intake to assess whether you're meeting your dietary needs. Pay attention to your intake of essential nutrients such as vitamins, minerals, protein, fiber, and healthy fats. Consider using a nutrition tracking app or consulting with a registered dietitian for a more detailed analysis.

Identify Food Patterns: Look for patterns or tendencies in your eating habits. Do you tend to skip meals or eat irregularly throughout the day? Are there certain types of foods that you gravitate towards or consume in excess? Identifying these patterns can help you understand your eating behavior and make targeted changes as needed.

Assess Portion Sizes: Take note of your portion sizes during meals and snacks. Are you consistently eating appropriate portion sizes, or do you tend to overeat? Pay attention to hunger and fullness cues to determine whether you're eating mindfully and stopping when satisfied.

Consider Emotional Eating: Reflect on whether your eating habits are influenced by emotions, stress, boredom, or other non-hunger-related factors. Do you turn to food for comfort or distraction? Recognizing emotional eating patterns can help you develop healthier coping strategies and establish a more balanced relationship with food.

Evaluate Meal Composition: Examine the composition of your meals to determine whether they are balanced and varied. Are you incorporating a variety of fruits, vegetables, whole grains, lean proteins, and healthy fats into your meals? Aim for a diverse and colorful plate to ensure you're getting a wide range of nutrients.

Reflect on Lifestyle Factors: Consider how factors such as work schedule, social activities, travel, and family responsibilities impact your eating habits. Are there specific challenges or obstacles that make it difficult to maintain a healthy diet? Identifying these barriers can help you develop strategies to overcome them and create a more sustainable eating plan.

By taking the time to assess your current eating habits, you can gain valuable insights into your dietary choices and behaviors. Armed with this information, you'll be better equipped to make informed decisions and set realistic goals for adopting a flexitarian approach to eating. Remember that change takes time, so be patient with yourself and celebrate progress along the way.

Setting Realistic Goals

When transitioning to a flexitarian diet or making any significant dietary changes, setting realistic goals is crucial for long-term success.

Here are some steps to help you establish achievable goals:

Define Your Objectives: Start by clarifying why you want to adopt a flexitarian lifestyle. Are you aiming to improve your health, reduce your environmental impact, or explore new culinary experiences? Identifying your motivations will help you set meaningful and relevant goals.

Be Specific: Rather than setting vague goals like "eat more plant-based foods," be specific about what you want to accomplish. For example, you could set a goal to consume at least five servings of fruits and vegetables per day or to replace one meat-based meal with a plant-based meal each week.

Gradual Progression: Instead of attempting drastic changes overnight, aim for gradual progression. Set small, achievable goals that you can build upon over time. For example, start by incorporating one meatless meal into your weekly menu and gradually increase the frequency as you become more comfortable with plant-based cooking.

Consider Your Lifestyle: Take into account your lifestyle, preferences, and dietary habits when setting goals. If you have a busy schedule or limited cooking skills, setting unrealistic goals like cooking elaborate plant-based meals every day may not be sustainable. Instead, focus on practical and achievable changes that align with your lifestyle.

Set SMART Goals: Use the SMART criteria to ensure your goals are Specific, Measurable, Achievable, Relevant, and Time-bound. For example, a SMART goal could be: "I will eat a plant-based lunch three days per week for the next month."

Monitor Your Progress: Keep track of your progress towards your goals and celebrate your successes along the way. Regularly assess how well you're sticking to your plan and make adjustments as needed. If you encounter challenges or setbacks, don't get discouraged—use them as learning opportunities to refine your approach.

Be Flexible: Flexibility is key to maintaining motivation and adapting to changing circumstances. If you find that certain goals are too challenging or no longer relevant, don't hesitate to modify them. Remember that the ultimate goal is progress, not perfection.

Focus on Non-Scale Victories: While weight loss or other measurable outcomes may be part of your goals, also focus on non-scale victories such as increased energy levels, improved mood, and enhanced culinary skills. These achievements can be just as meaningful and rewarding as tangible results.

By setting realistic and achievable goals, you can lay the foundation for long-term success in adopting a flexitarian lifestyle. Remember to approach the process with patience, perseverance, and a willingness to embrace change.

Stocking Your Kitchen for Success

Creating a well-equipped kitchen is essential for embracing a flexitarian lifestyle and making healthy, plant-based meals convenient and enjoyable. Here are some tips for stocking your kitchen for success:

Essential Pantry Staples

- **Whole grains:** Brown rice, quinoa, oats, whole wheat pasta
- **Legumes:** Lentils, chickpeas, black beans, kidney beans
- **Canned or dried fruits and vegetables:** Tomatoes, beans, corn, dried fruits

- **Nuts and seeds:** Almonds, walnuts, chia seeds, flaxseeds
- **Nut butters:** Peanut butter, almond butter, tahini
- **Herbs and spices:** Garlic, onion, basil, oregano, cumin, turmeric, cinnamon
- **Healthy oils:** Olive oil, coconut oil, avocado oil

Fresh Produce

- **Seasonal fruits and vegetables:** Stock up on a variety of fresh produce to incorporate into your meals. Aim for a colorful assortment to ensure a diverse range of nutrients.
- **Leafy greens:** Spinach, kale, arugula, lettuce
- **Cruciferous vegetables:** Broccoli, cauliflower, Brussels sprouts
- **Root vegetables:** Carrots, sweet potatoes, beets

- **Fresh herbs:** Parsley, cilantro, mint, basil

Plant-Based Proteins

- **Tofu:** Firm tofu can be marinated and used in stir-fries, salads, or grilled dishes.

- **Tempeh:** A fermented soy product with a nutty flavor, great for adding protein to salads, sandwiches, and stir-fries.

- **Seitan:** A high-protein meat substitute made from wheat gluten, ideal for hearty dishes like stews and roasts.

- **Plant-based burgers and sausages:** Keep a supply of frozen plant-based burgers and sausages on hand for quick and convenient meals.

Dairy and Dairy Alternatives

- **Non-dairy milk:** Stock up on options like almond milk, soy milk, oat milk, or coconut milk for use in smoothies, cereal, and cooking.

- **Yogurt alternatives:** Choose from a variety of non-dairy yogurts made from almond, coconut, or soy milk.

- **Cheese alternatives:** Explore different brands and types of plant-based cheeses made from nuts, soy, or tapioca starch.

Whole Foods Snacks

- **Fresh fruit:** Keep a bowl of fresh fruit on the countertop for easy snacking.

- **Raw vegetables:** Wash and chop vegetables like carrots, celery, and bell peppers for quick, healthy snacks.

- **Whole grain crackers and rice cakes:** Choose whole grain options for a satisfying crunch.

- **Hummus and guacamole:** Keep containers of hummus and guacamole on hand for dipping vegetables or spreading on whole grain toast.

Kitchen Tools and Equipment

- **Blender or food processor:** Essential for making smoothies, sauces, dips, and soups.

- **Quality knives and cutting boards:** Invest in sharp knives and durable cutting boards for safe and efficient meal preparation.

- **Non-stick cookware:** Choose non-stick pots and pans for easy cooking and cleaning, especially when preparing plant-based meals that may not contain added oils.

- **Baking essentials:** Stock up on baking pans, mixing bowls, measuring cups, and utensils for making homemade bread, muffins, and other baked goods.

By stocking your kitchen with a variety of plant-based ingredients, protein sources, dairy alternatives, and essential kitchen tools, you'll be well-prepared to embrace a flexitarian lifestyle and create delicious, nutritious meals at home. Experiment with new recipes, flavors, and ingredients to keep your meals exciting and satisfying.

CHAPTER 2
THE FOUNDATION: PLANT-BASED NUTRITION
The Power of Plants: Nutritional Benefits

Plants are nutritional powerhouses, packed with a wide array of vitamins, minerals, antioxidants, and phytonutrients that promote health and well-being. Here's a closer look at the nutritional benefits of incorporating more plant-based foods into your diet:

Abundance of Nutrients: Plant-based foods provide essential nutrients that are vital for overall health, including vitamins A, C, E, and K, as well as folate, potassium, magnesium, and fiber. By consuming a variety of fruits, vegetables, whole grains, legumes, nuts, and seeds, you can ensure you're getting a diverse range of nutrients to support various bodily functions.

Rich in Antioxidants: Many plant foods are rich in antioxidants, compounds that help protect cells from damage caused by harmful molecules called free radicals. Antioxidants play a key role in reducing inflammation, boosting immune function, and preventing chronic diseases such as heart disease, cancer, and neurodegenerative disorders. Berries, leafy greens, nuts, seeds, and brightly colored fruits and vegetables are particularly high in antioxidants.

High in Fiber: Plant-based foods are excellent sources of dietary fiber, which is essential for digestive health, weight management, and reducing the risk of chronic diseases such as diabetes and heart disease. Fiber helps promote satiety, regulate blood sugar levels, and support a healthy gut microbiome by feeding beneficial bacteria in the digestive tract. Whole grains, legumes, fruits, vegetables, and nuts are all rich sources of fiber.

Lower in Saturated Fat and Cholesterol: Compared to animal-based foods, plant-based foods are generally lower in saturated fat and cholesterol, making them heart-healthy choices. Diets high in saturated fat and cholesterol have been linked to an increased risk of heart disease and stroke, whereas plant-based diets have been associated with lower cholesterol levels and improved cardiovascular health.

Reduced Risk of Chronic Diseases: Numerous studies have shown that plant-based diets are associated with a lower risk of chronic diseases such as heart disease, diabetes, obesity, and certain types of cancer. The abundance of nutrients, fiber, and antioxidants found in plant foods can help reduce inflammation, lower blood pressure and cholesterol levels, and support overall health and longevity.

Environmental Sustainability: In addition to their nutritional benefits, plant-based diets are also more environmentally sustainable compared to diets rich in animal products. Plant foods require fewer natural resources, such as water and land, and produce fewer greenhouse gas emissions, making them more eco-friendly choices. By reducing meat consumption and incorporating more plant-based foods into your diet, you can contribute to environmental conservation efforts and help mitigate climate change.

Incorporating a variety of plant-based foods into your diet can provide a wealth of nutritional benefits that support overall health, longevity, and environmental sustainability. Aim to fill your plate with a colorful assortment of fruits, vegetables, whole grains, legumes, nuts, and seeds to reap the full spectrum of nutrients and phytonutrients that plants have to offer.

Building Balanced Meals without Meat

Creating balanced and satisfying meals without meat is not only feasible but also offers numerous health benefits. By incorporating a variety of plant-based foods, you can ensure you're getting all the essential nutrients your body needs. Here's how to build balanced meat-free meals:

Start with Plant-Based Protein Sources
Legumes: Beans, lentils, chickpeas, and peas are excellent sources of protein, fiber, and various vitamins and minerals. Incorporate them into soups, stews, salads, and wraps for a hearty and nutritious meal.

Tofu and Tempeh: These soy-based products are versatile protein sources that can be marinated, grilled, stir-fried, or baked. Use them in place of meat in dishes like stir-fries, curries, and sandwiches.

Quinoa and Other Whole Grains: Whole grains like quinoa, brown rice, barley, and farro are not only rich in protein but also provide fiber, vitamins, and minerals. Use them as a base for grain bowls, salads, and pilafs.

Nuts and Seeds: Incorporate nuts and seeds such as almonds, walnuts, chia seeds, and hemp seeds into your meals for added protein, healthy fats, and crunch. Sprinkle them on salads, yogurt, oatmeal, or use them as a topping for roasted vegetables.

Load Up on Vegetables
Fill half your plate with a variety of colorful vegetables to ensure you're getting a wide range of nutrients. Opt for leafy greens like spinach, kale, and Swiss chard, as well as cruciferous vegetables like broccoli, cauliflower, and Brussels sprouts.

Include a mix of raw and cooked vegetables to add texture and flavor to your meals. Roast vegetables with herbs and spices for a caramelized sweetness, or enjoy them raw with hummus or yogurt-based dips.

Experiment with different cooking methods such as steaming, sautéing, grilling, and stir-frying to bring out the natural flavors of vegetables while retaining their nutrients.

Add Healthy Fats

Incorporate sources of healthy fats such as avocados, olives, nuts, seeds, and olive oil into your meals to promote satiety and enhance flavor. Avocado slices make a delicious addition to salads, sandwiches, and wraps, while drizzling olive oil over roasted vegetables adds richness and depth of flavor.

Choose unsaturated fats over saturated fats and trans fats to support heart health. Foods like avocado, nuts, seeds, and olive oil are rich in monounsaturated and polyunsaturated fats, which have been shown to lower cholesterol levels and reduce the risk of heart disease.

Don't Forget About Calcium and Vitamin D
While dairy products are common sources of calcium and vitamin D, you can also find these nutrients in plant-based foods. Opt for fortified plant milks such as almond, soy, or oat milk, and choose calcium-rich foods like tofu, tempeh, fortified cereals, leafy greens, and calcium-set tofu.

Flavor with Herbs, Spices, and Sauces
Enhance the flavor of your meat-free meals with a variety of herbs, spices, and sauces. Experiment with different flavor combinations to keep your meals exciting and enjoyable. Fresh herbs like basil, cilantro, mint, and parsley add brightness and freshness to dishes, while spices like cumin, paprika, turmeric, and curry powder add depth and complexity.

Building balanced meals without meat is not only nutritious but also delicious and satisfying. By incorporating a variety of plant-based protein sources, vegetables, healthy fats, and flavor-enhancing ingredients, you can create flavorful and nourishing meals that support your health and well-being. Experiment with different ingredients and recipes to discover new favorites and enjoy the benefits of a plant-centric diet.

Exploring a Variety of Plant-Based Proteins

Plant-based proteins offer a diverse and nutritious alternative to meat, providing essential amino acids, vitamins, minerals, and other health-promoting nutrients. Here's a guide to exploring the wide range of plant-based protein sources and incorporating them into your diet:

Legumes

Beans: Black beans, kidney beans, chickpeas, lentils, and navy beans are versatile and affordable sources of plant-based protein. They can be used in a variety of dishes, including soups, stews, salads, and tacos.

Lentils: Rich in protein, fiber, and iron, lentils come in various colors and varieties, including green, red, and black. They cook quickly and can be used as a meat substitute in recipes like vegetarian burgers, meatloaf, and sloppy joes.

Tofu and Tempeh

Tofu: Made from soybeans, tofu is a versatile and protein-rich ingredient that absorbs flavors well. It comes in different textures, including silken, soft, firm, and extra-firm, making it suitable for various dishes like stir-fries, curries, scrambles, and smoothies.

Tempeh: A fermented soybean product, tempeh has a nutty flavor and firm texture. It's a good source of protein, probiotics, and fiber, making it ideal for grilling, baking, or crumbling into salads, sandwiches, and stir-fries.

Whole Grains

Quinoa: Often referred to as a "complete protein," quinoa contains all nine essential amino acids, making it an excellent plant-based protein source. It's versatile and can be used in salads, pilafs, stir-fries, and breakfast bowls.

Brown Rice: Brown rice is a whole grain that provides protein, fiber, and essential nutrients like magnesium and selenium. It can be paired with beans, tofu, or vegetables in dishes like rice bowls, stir-fries, and stuffed peppers.

Nuts and Seeds

Almonds: Almonds are rich in protein, healthy fats, fiber, and antioxidants. Enjoy them as a snack, sprinkle them on salads or oatmeal, or use them to make almond butter or almond milk.

Chia Seeds: Chia seeds are packed with protein, fiber, omega-3 fatty acids, and calcium. They can be added to smoothies, yogurt, oatmeal, or used to make chia pudding.

Hemp Seeds: Hemp seeds are a complete protein source containing all nine essential amino acids. They're nutty in flavor and can be sprinkled on salads, soups, or blended into smoothies.

Plant-Based Meat Alternatives

Plant-based burgers: Made from ingredients like peas, soy, or mushrooms, plant-based burgers mimic the taste and texture of traditional meat burgers. They're widely available in grocery stores and can be grilled, baked, or pan-fried.

Veggie sausages: These meatless sausages are typically made from a combination of vegetables, grains, and spices. They can be grilled, roasted, or sautéed and served alongside vegetables, pasta, or grains.

Incorporating a variety of plant-based protein sources into your diet ensures you're getting a diverse array of nutrients while supporting your health, the environment, and animal welfare. Experiment with different ingredients and recipes to discover new flavors and enjoy the benefits of a plant-centric diet.

CHAPTER 3
INCORPORATING ANIMAL PRODUCTS MINDFULLY

Understanding the Role of Animal Products in a Flexitarian Diet

In a flexitarian diet, the consumption of animal products is approached with mindfulness and moderation. While the primary focus is on plant-based foods, the occasional inclusion of animal products can provide certain nutrients and flavor profiles that contribute to a varied and balanced diet. Here's a closer look at the role of animal products in a flexitarian diet:

Nutrient Contribution: Animal products, such as meat, poultry, fish, eggs, and dairy, are rich sources of essential nutrients such as protein, vitamin B12, iron, zinc, and omega-3 fatty acids. Including small servings of these foods in a flexitarian diet can help ensure you're meeting your nutritional needs, particularly for nutrients that may be less abundant in plant-based foods.

Protein Quality: Animal-based proteins are considered complete proteins, meaning they contain all nine essential amino acids that the body cannot produce on its own. While plant-based proteins can also be nutritious and provide essential amino acids, some may be lower in certain amino acids. By incorporating small amounts of animal products into a flexitarian diet, you can enhance the overall protein quality of your meals.

Flavor and Texture: Animal products often contribute distinct flavors, textures, and mouthfeel to dishes that can enhance the overall eating experience. Whether it's the umami richness of meat, the creaminess of dairy products, or the flakiness of fish, incorporating animal products can add variety and enjoyment to meals, making it easier to maintain a balanced and satisfying diet.

Cultural and Social Considerations: For many individuals, animal products play a significant role in cultural traditions, family gatherings, and social events. Embracing a flexitarian approach allows for flexibility in navigating different food environments and social situations while still honoring cultural and personal preferences. By including small amounts of animal products on occasion, flexitarians can participate in shared meals and cultural celebrations without feeling restricted by dietary choices.

Environmental and Ethical Awareness: While animal products can provide valuable nutrients and flavor, their production also has environmental and ethical implications. Industrial animal agriculture is associated with issues such as deforestation, water pollution, greenhouse gas emissions, and animal welfare concerns. By reducing overall meat consumption and choosing sustainably sourced and ethically raised animal products when they are included, flexitarians can minimize their environmental footprint and support more humane farming practices.

In summary, the role of animal products in a flexitarian diet is one of balance, mindfulness, and moderation. While plant-based foods form the foundation of the diet, the occasional inclusion of animal products can provide nutritional benefits, enhance culinary diversity, and accommodate cultural and social preferences. By adopting a flexible and conscious approach to food choices, flexitarians can enjoy the best of both worlds—nourishing their bodies while minimizing their impact on the planet and respecting ethical considerations.

Choosing Quality Over Quantity: Selecting Sustainable and Ethical Options

In a flexitarian diet, prioritizing quality over quantity when it comes to selecting animal products is key to supporting sustainability and ethical practices. By making conscious choices about where and how your food is sourced, you can reduce your environmental impact, support humane treatment of animals, and promote overall well-being. Here are some guidelines for selecting sustainable and ethical options:

Know Your Sources: Take the time to research and understand where your food comes from. Choose products from local farms and producers that prioritize sustainable farming practices, animal welfare, and environmental stewardship. Look for certifications such as Certified Organic, Animal

Welfare Approved, and Certified Humane to ensure higher standards of production.

Opt for Pasture-Raised and Grass-Fed: When selecting animal products such as meat, poultry, and dairy, choose options that are pasture-raised and grass-fed whenever possible. Animals raised in pasture-based systems have access to open space, fresh air, and natural grazing, resulting in healthier animals and more nutrient-dense products. Look for labels like "Pasture-Raised," "Grass-Fed," or "Certified Organic" to identify these products.

Support Sustainable Seafood: If you consume fish and seafood, opt for sustainably sourced options that are harvested using environmentally responsible practices. Look for certifications such as Marine Stewardship Council (MSC) or Aquaculture Stewardship Council (ASC) to ensure that the seafood you choose is caught or farmed in a way that minimizes harm to marine ecosystems and supports the long-term health of fish populations.

Choose Organic and Non-GMO: Whenever possible, choose organic and non-GMO (genetically modified organism) options to minimize exposure to pesticides, herbicides, and genetically engineered ingredients. Organic farming practices promote soil health, biodiversity, and ecological balance while reducing the use of synthetic chemicals and minimizing environmental impact.

Reduce Food Waste: Another aspect of choosing quality over quantity is minimizing food waste. Plan meals thoughtfully, use leftovers creatively, and store perishable items properly to extend their shelf life. By reducing food waste, you can make the most of the resources that went into producing your food and minimize your ecological footprint.

Consider Plant-Based Alternatives: In addition to selecting high-quality animal products, consider incorporating more plant-based alternatives into your diet. Plant-based proteins such as tofu, tempeh, lentils, and beans can provide nutritious and delicious alternatives to meat, poultry, and dairy products while reducing the environmental impact of your diet.

Support Local and Sustainable Agriculture: Whenever possible, support local farmers, farmers' markets, and community-supported agriculture (CSA) programs that prioritize sustainable farming practices, soil health, and biodiversity. Buying directly from local producers not only ensures fresher, more flavorful foods but also strengthens local food systems and reduces the carbon footprint associated with transportation.

By choosing quality over quantity and selecting sustainable and ethical options, you can make a positive impact on your health, the environment, and the welfare of animals. By supporting producers who prioritize sustainability, you can contribute to a more resilient and equitable food system while enjoying delicious and nourishing meals.

Portion Control and Moderation Guidelines

In a flexitarian diet, portion control and moderation are essential principles for maintaining balance, preventing overconsumption, and optimizing health. While flexibility is a hallmark of the flexitarian approach, mindful eating practices can help ensure that you're meeting your nutritional needs while enjoying a diverse range of foods.

Here are some portion control and moderation guidelines to consider:

Listen to Your Body: Pay attention to your body's hunger and fullness cues to guide your portion sizes. Eat when you're hungry and stop when you're satisfied, aiming for a comfortable level of fullness without feeling overly stuffed. Avoid mindless eating and distractions such as watching TV or scrolling on your phone, which can lead to overeating.

Practice Mindful Eating: Take the time to savor and enjoy your meals, focusing on the flavors, textures, and aromas of the food. Chew slowly and mindfully, allowing yourself to fully experience each bite. By eating mindfully, you'll be more in tune with your body's signals of hunger and fullness, making it easier to gauge appropriate portion sizes.

Use Visual Cues: Use visual cues to help estimate appropriate portion sizes. For example, a serving of protein (such as meat, poultry, or fish) should be about the size of your palm, while a serving of grains or starches (such as rice, pasta, or potatoes) should be about the size of your fist. Fill the rest of your plate with non-starchy vegetables to add volume and nutrients without excess calories.

Be Mindful of Caloric Density: Be mindful of the caloric density of different foods and adjust your portions accordingly. High-calorie foods such as nuts, seeds, oils, and dairy products should be enjoyed in moderation to avoid excess calorie intake. Incorporate these foods into your meals mindfully and consider smaller portion sizes to balance your overall energy intake.

Include a Variety of Foods: Aim for a balanced and varied diet by including a wide range of foods from different food groups. Incorporate plenty of fruits, vegetables, whole grains, legumes, nuts, seeds, and lean proteins into your meals to ensure you're getting a diverse array of nutrients. Experiment with different flavors, textures, and cuisines to keep your meals interesting and satisfying.

Be Flexible: Flexibility is a key principle of the flexitarian diet, so don't be too rigid or restrictive with your portion sizes. Allow yourself to enjoy occasional indulgences or treats without guilt, but aim to balance them out with healthier choices throughout the day. It's all about finding a sustainable and balanced approach that works for you.

Pay Attention to Serving Sizes: Familiarize yourself with standard serving sizes for different foods to help guide your portion control. Use measuring cups, spoons, or kitchen scales to accurately portion out foods, especially when cooking or preparing meals at home. Over time, you'll develop a better sense of appropriate portion sizes based on your individual needs and preferences.

By practicing portion control and moderation, you can enjoy the flexibility and variety of a flexitarian diet while maintaining balance and optimizing your health. Remember to listen to your body, eat mindfully, and make conscious choices that align with your nutritional goals and preferences. With practice and patience, portion control can become a natural and intuitive part of your eating habits.

CHAPTER 4
FLEXITARIAN RECIPES FOR EVERY OCCASION
Breakfast Delights: Energizing Starters

Starting your day with a nutritious and energizing breakfast sets the tone for a day of healthy eating and sustained energy. Here are some breakfast ideas to kickstart your morning and fuel your day:

Smoothie Bowls: Blend together your favorite fruits, leafy greens, and plant-based milk or yogurt to create a thick and creamy smoothie base. Pour the smoothie into a bowl and top it with a variety of toppings such as fresh fruit slices, granola, nuts, seeds, and coconut flakes for added texture, flavor, and nutrition.

Overnight Oats: Combine rolled oats with your choice of milk (dairy or plant-based) in a jar or container, along with toppings like chia seeds, sliced fruit, nuts, and a drizzle of honey or maple syrup. Let the mixture sit in the refrigerator overnight, and in the morning, you'll have a delicious and convenient breakfast ready to enjoy, either cold or warmed up.

Avocado Toast: Mash ripe avocado onto whole grain toast and top it with sliced tomatoes, a sprinkle of sea salt, and a drizzle of olive oil for a simple yet satisfying breakfast. For added protein and flavor, top your avocado toast with a poached or fried egg, smoked salmon, or crumbled feta cheese.

Veggie Omelette: Whisk together eggs or tofu with diced vegetables such as bell peppers, onions, spinach, mushrooms, and tomatoes. Cook the mixture in a non-stick skillet until set, then fold it over to create a fluffy omelette. Serve with a side of whole grain toast or a handful of mixed berries for a balanced and nutritious meal.

Greek Yogurt Parfait: Layer Greek yogurt with fresh berries, sliced fruit, granola, and a drizzle of honey or maple syrup in a glass or bowl to create a colorful and satisfying parfait. Greek yogurt is rich in protein and probiotics, while the fruits and granola add sweetness, fiber, and crunch.

Breakfast Burritos: Fill whole grain tortillas with scrambled eggs or tofu, black beans, diced avocado, salsa, and shredded cheese for a hearty and portable breakfast option. Wrap the burritos tightly and enjoy them on the go or pack them for a quick and convenient meal at work or school.

Chia Seed Pudding: Mix chia seeds with your choice of milk (such as almond, coconut, or soy milk) and a touch of sweetener (like honey, maple syrup, or agave nectar). Let the mixture sit in the refrigerator for a few hours or overnight until thickened, then top it with fresh fruit, nuts, and a sprinkle of cinnamon for a nutritious and satisfying pudding-like breakfast.

These breakfast delights are not only delicious and satisfying but also packed with essential nutrients to fuel your body and brain for a productive day ahead. Experiment with different flavors, ingredients, and combinations to find your favorite breakfast starters and make mornings something to look forward to.

Flavorful Lunches: Plant-Powered Creations

Lunchtime offers the perfect opportunity to refuel your body with nutritious and satisfying plant-powered meals. Whether you're packing lunch for work or enjoying a midday meal at home, here are some flavorful lunch ideas that celebrate the vibrant flavors and versatility of plant-based ingredients:

Quinoa Salad with Roasted Vegetables: Toss cooked quinoa with a variety of roasted vegetables such as bell peppers, zucchini, eggplant, cherry tomatoes, and red onions. Drizzle with a tangy balsamic vinaigrette and sprinkle with fresh herbs like basil or parsley for a colorful and nutritious salad that's both hearty and satisfying.

Buddha Bowl: Build a nourishing Buddha bowl by combining cooked grains (such as brown rice, farro, or barley) with a variety of colorful vegetables, legumes, and greens. Add roasted sweet potatoes, steamed broccoli, sautéed kale, avocado slices, chickpeas, and a dollop of tahini or hummus for a balanced and flavorful meal in a bowl.

Stuffed Bell Peppers: Fill halved bell peppers with a mixture of cooked quinoa or rice, black beans, corn, diced tomatoes, onions, and spices such as cumin, chili powder, and paprika. Top with shredded vegan cheese or avocado slices, then bake until the peppers are tender and the filling is heated through for a delicious and satisfying stuffed pepper dish.

Veggie Wrap with Hummus: Spread a whole grain wrap with a generous layer of hummus, then fill it with an assortment of thinly sliced vegetables such as cucumbers, bell peppers, carrots, spinach, and avocado. Roll up the wrap tightly and slice it in half for a portable and nutritious lunch option that's packed with flavor and fiber.

Mediterranean Salad with Falafel: Assemble a Mediterranean-inspired salad with mixed greens, cherry tomatoes, cucumber slices, red onion, olives, and crumbled vegan feta cheese. Top the salad with crispy homemade or store-bought falafel balls and drizzle with a lemon-tahini dressing for a satisfying and protein-rich lunch.

Lentil Soup with Crusty Bread: Simmer lentils with diced vegetables, vegetable broth, and aromatic spices like garlic, cumin, and thyme to create a hearty and comforting lentil soup. Serve the soup with crusty whole grain bread for dipping, or pair it with a side salad for a complete and nourishing meal that's perfect for cooler days.

Sushi Bowl: Deconstruct your favorite sushi roll and transform it into a colorful and flavorful sushi bowl. Start with a base of sushi rice or brown rice, then top it with sliced avocado, cucumber, carrots, edamame, and seaweed strips. Drizzle with soy sauce, sriracha, and sesame seeds for added flavor, and enjoy a taste of sushi without the fuss of rolling.

These plant-powered lunch creations are not only delicious and satisfying but also packed with nutrients to keep you feeling energized and focused throughout the day. Experiment with different ingredients, flavors, and textures to create your own plant-based masterpieces and enjoy the benefits of a vibrant and nourishing midday meal.

Wholesome Dinners: Satisfying and Nourishing Meals

After a long day, there's nothing quite like sitting down to a satisfying and nourishing dinner. Whether you're cooking for yourself, your family, or friends, dinner offers an opportunity to unwind, connect, and refuel your body with wholesome foods. Here are some ideas for creating delicious and nutritious dinners that are sure to please:

Vegetable Stir-Fry: Stir-fries are quick, versatile, and perfect for using up any leftover vegetables in your fridge. Heat a wok or large skillet over high heat and stir-fry a colorful array of vegetables such as bell peppers, broccoli, snap peas, carrots, and mushrooms. Add tofu, tempeh, or edamame for protein, and season with a savory sauce made from soy sauce, garlic, ginger, and sesame oil. Serve over cooked brown rice or noodles for a satisfying and well-balanced meal.

Lentil Shepherd's Pie: This comforting and hearty dish is a plant-based twist on the classic shepherd's pie. Simmer lentils with onions, garlic, carrots, and celery in vegetable broth until tender, then top with a layer of creamy mashed potatoes or mashed cauliflower. Bake until golden and bubbly for a wholesome and satisfying dinner that's perfect for chilly evenings.

Chickpea Curry with Coconut Rice: This flavorful and aromatic curry is made with tender chickpeas simmered in a rich and creamy coconut sauce. Add diced tomatoes, onions, garlic, ginger, and spices like curry powder, turmeric, and cumin for depth of flavor. Serve the curry over fragrant coconut rice garnished with chopped cilantro and a squeeze of lime for a delicious and satisfying meal that's sure to please.

Portobello Mushroom Burgers: Grilled portobello mushrooms make a delicious and hearty alternative to meat burgers. Marinate the mushrooms in a mixture of balsamic vinegar, soy sauce, garlic, and olive oil, then grill until tender and charred. Serve the mushrooms on whole grain buns with your favorite burger toppings such as lettuce, tomato, avocado, and caramelized onions for a wholesome and satisfying dinner that's perfect for summer cookouts.

Spaghetti Squash Primavera: Swap traditional pasta for spaghetti squash in this lighter and lower-carb version of classic pasta primavera. Roast spaghetti squash until tender, then use a fork to scrape out the strands. Toss the squash with sautéed vegetables such as cherry tomatoes, zucchini, bell peppers, and spinach in a garlic-infused olive oil sauce. Finish with a sprinkle of grated Parmesan cheese or nutritional yeast for a satisfying and veggie-packed meal.

Stuffed Bell Peppers with Quinoa and Black Beans: These colorful and nutritious bell peppers are filled with a hearty mixture of cooked quinoa, black beans, corn, onions, and spices. Top with shredded vegan cheese or avocado slices and bake until the peppers are tender and the filling is heated through. Serve with a side of salsa or guacamole for a flavorful and protein-rich dinner that's perfect for Meatless Mondays.

Veggie-packed Pizza: Homemade pizza is a fun and customizable way to pack in plenty of vegetables and flavor. Start with a whole wheat or cauliflower pizza crust, then top it with tomato sauce, shredded mozzarella cheese or dairy-free cheese, and a variety of colorful vegetables such as bell peppers, onions, mushrooms, spinach, and olives. Bake until the crust is golden and crispy, then garnish with fresh basil or arugula for a satisfying and veggie-loaded meal.

These wholesome dinner ideas are just a starting point for creating delicious and nourishing meals that you and your loved ones will enjoy. Feel free to get creative and adapt these recipes to suit your tastes and dietary preferences, and don't forget to savor the mealtime experience and enjoy the company of those around you.

Snacks and Sides: Tasty Bites for Anytime Cravings

Whether you're looking for a mid-afternoon pick-me-up or a flavorful accompaniment to your main meals, having a selection of tasty snacks and sides on hand is essential. Here are some delicious and nutritious options to satisfy your cravings anytime:

Veggie Sticks with Hummus: Crunchy raw vegetables such as carrot sticks, cucumber slices, bell pepper strips, and celery sticks pair perfectly with creamy hummus for a satisfying and nutritious snack. The combination of fiber-rich veggies and protein-packed hummus makes this a satisfying option that will keep you feeling full and energized.

Trail Mix: Create your own custom trail mix by combining a variety of nuts, seeds, dried fruits, and whole grain cereal or pretzels. Choose unsalted nuts and seeds for a healthier option, and mix in dried fruits like raisins, apricots, and cranberries for a touch of natural sweetness. Trail mix is perfect for on-the-go snacking and provides a mix of protein, healthy fats, and carbohydrates to keep you fueled throughout the day.

Guacamole with Whole Grain Crackers: Creamy and flavorful guacamole made from ripe avocados, lime juice, garlic, cilantro, and diced tomatoes is perfect for dipping whole grain crackers or baked tortilla chips. Avocados are rich in heart-healthy monounsaturated fats and fiber, making guacamole a nutritious and satisfying snack option.

Roasted Chickpeas: Crispy roasted chickpeas seasoned with your favorite spices make a delicious and protein-packed snack. Simply toss cooked chickpeas with olive oil and spices such as paprika, cumin, garlic powder, and cayenne pepper, then roast in the oven until golden and crunchy. Enjoy roasted chickpeas on their own or as a crunchy topping for salads and soups.

Greek Yogurt Parfait: Layer creamy Greek yogurt with fresh berries, sliced fruit, granola, and a drizzle of honey or maple syrup for a delicious and nutritious parfait. Greek yogurt is high in protein and probiotics, while the fruits and granola add fiber, vitamins, and minerals. Enjoy a Greek yogurt parfait as a satisfying snack or a light dessert option.

Veggie Chips: Make your own crispy veggie chips by thinly slicing vegetables such as sweet potatoes, beets, carrots, or zucchini, then baking or air-frying until crispy. Season with a sprinkle of salt, pepper, and your favorite herbs or spices for a flavorful and crunchy snack that's perfect for munching on anytime.

Caprese Skewers: Skewer cherry tomatoes, fresh mozzarella balls, and basil leaves on toothpicks or skewers for a simple and elegant snack or appetizer. Drizzle with balsamic glaze and a sprinkle of sea salt and black pepper for added flavor. Caprese skewers are perfect for entertaining or enjoying as a light and refreshing snack.

These tasty bites for anytime cravings are not only delicious and satisfying but also packed with nutrients to fuel your body and keep you feeling energized throughout the day. Whether you're looking for a quick snack on the go or a flavorful side to accompany your meals, these options are sure to hit the spot. Feel free to get creative and customize these snacks and sides to suit your tastes and dietary preferences.

Indulgent Treats: Desserts to Satisfy Your Sweet Tooth

Sometimes, nothing quite hits the spot like a delicious dessert to satisfy your sweet cravings. Whether you're celebrating a special occasion or simply treating yourself, here are some indulgent dessert ideas that are sure to delight:

Decadent Chocolate Brownies: Rich, fudgy chocolate brownies are a classic dessert that never fails to satisfy. Whether you prefer them plain, studded with nuts, or swirled with caramel or peanut butter, there's a brownie recipe to suit every taste. Serve warm with a scoop of vanilla ice cream for an extra indulgent treat.

Creamy Cheesecake: Smooth and creamy cheesecake is a luxurious dessert that's perfect for special occasions. Whether you prefer classic New York-style cheesecake, fruity variations like strawberry or raspberry swirl, or decadent chocolate cheesecake, there's a flavor for everyone. Top with fresh fruit, whipped cream, or chocolate ganache for added flair.

Classic Chocolate Chip Cookies: Soft and chewy chocolate chip cookies are a beloved treat that never goes out of style. Whether you enjoy them warm from the oven or dunked in a glass of milk, there's something irresistible about a freshly baked chocolate chip cookie. Experiment with different variations like adding nuts, oats, or coconut for added texture and flavor.

Decadent Chocolate Truffles: Rich and indulgent chocolate truffles are perfect for satisfying your sweet tooth with just a few luxurious bites. Made with a mixture of chocolate, cream, and butter, these velvety smooth confections can be rolled in cocoa powder, chopped nuts, or shredded coconut for an extra layer of flavor and texture.

Silky Panna Cotta: Elegant and sophisticated, panna cotta is a creamy Italian dessert that's surprisingly simple to make. Made with a mixture of cream, milk, sugar, and gelatin, panna cotta can be flavored with vanilla, coffee, chocolate, or fruit puree for endless variations. Serve chilled with a drizzle of fruit compote or caramel sauce for a stunning presentation.

Decadent Chocolate Mousse: Light and airy chocolate mousse is a luxurious dessert that's perfect for special occasions. Made with whipped cream, egg whites, and melted chocolate, chocolate mousse is rich, indulgent, and irresistibly smooth. Serve in individual glasses or ramekins and garnish with whipped cream and chocolate shavings for an elegant finishing touch.

Fruit Tart with Vanilla Custard: Fresh fruit tart topped with vanilla custard is a delightful dessert that showcases the beauty of seasonal fruits. Start with a buttery tart crust, fill it with creamy vanilla custard, and top with an assortment of sliced fruit such as berries, kiwi, peaches, and grapes. Brush with apricot glaze for a glossy finish and serve chilled for a refreshing and indulgent treat.

These indulgent dessert ideas are perfect for satisfying your sweet tooth and treating yourself to something special. Whether you prefer rich and chocolatey treats, creamy and decadent desserts, or fruity and refreshing options, there's something here for everyone to enjoy. So go ahead, indulge a little, and savor every delicious bite!

CHAPTER 5
NAVIGATING SOCIAL SITUATIONS AND EATING OUT

Communicating Your Dietary Choices Effectively

Effectively communicating your dietary choices is important for fostering understanding, respect, and support from others, whether it's family members, friends, coworkers, or restaurant staff. Here are some strategies to help you communicate your dietary choices effectively:

Be Confident and Clear: When discussing your dietary choices with others, be confident and clear about your reasons for following a particular diet. Whether you're vegetarian, vegan, flexitarian, or following a specific eating plan for health or ethical reasons, clearly communicate your preferences and boundaries without apologizing or feeling the need to justify yourself.

Educate Others: Take the opportunity to educate others about your dietary choices and the reasons behind them. Share information about the health benefits, environmental impact, or ethical considerations associated with your chosen diet in a non-confrontational and informative manner. By providing context and perspective, you can help others better understand and respect your choices.

Offer Solutions: When dining out or attending social gatherings, offer solutions or alternatives to accommodate your dietary preferences. For example, suggest restaurants that offer vegetarian or vegan options, offer to bring a dish to share that aligns with your diet, or communicate your needs to the host in advance so they can plan accordingly. By being proactive and flexible, you can help ensure that everyone can enjoy the meal together.

Lead by Example: Instead of preaching or lecturing others about your dietary choices, lead by example and let your actions speak for themselves. Show others how delicious, satisfying, and fulfilling your chosen diet can be by sharing your favorite recipes, meals, and snacks. Be open to answering questions and providing guidance to those who are curious or interested in learning more.

Respect Differences: Remember that not everyone shares the same dietary beliefs or preferences as you, and that's okay. Respect the dietary choices of others, even if they differ from your own, and avoid judgment or criticism. Instead, focus on finding common ground and mutual respect, and celebrate the diversity of food choices and perspectives.

Be Flexible: While it's important to communicate your dietary choices effectively, it's also important to be flexible and adaptable in certain situations. Recognize that there may be times when you need to compromise or make exceptions, such as when dining at a restaurant with limited options or attending a special event. Be open to finding creative solutions and making the best choices available to you in any given situation.

Seek Support: Surround yourself with supportive individuals who respect and understand your dietary choices. Whether it's joining a community of like-minded individuals, seeking support from friends and family members, or connecting with online forums and social media groups, having a support network can help reinforce your commitment to your chosen diet and provide encouragement along the way.

By effectively communicating your dietary choices with confidence, clarity, and respect, you can foster understanding, build support, and navigate social situations with ease. Remember to be patient, open-minded, and flexible, and focus on finding common ground and mutual respect in your interactions with others.

Strategies for Dining Out as a Flexitarian

Dining out as a flexitarian can present unique challenges and opportunities, as you navigate menus to find options that align with your primarily plant-based diet while still allowing for occasional inclusion of meat or other animal products. Here are some strategies to help you enjoy dining out while staying true to your flexitarian lifestyle:

Research Restaurants in Advance: Before heading out to eat, take some time to research restaurants in your area that offer a variety of plant-based options as well as dishes that include meat or other animal products. Look for eateries that prioritize fresh, seasonal ingredients and are known for accommodating dietary preferences and restrictions.

Scan the Menu Carefully: When you arrive at the restaurant, carefully scan the menu for dishes that can be easily customized to suit your flexitarian diet. Look for options that feature plenty of vegetables, grains, legumes, and plant-based proteins, and consider asking if meat can be added or substituted on certain dishes if you're in the mood for it.

Don't Be Afraid to Ask Questions: If you're unsure about the ingredients or preparation methods of a particular dish, don't hesitate to ask your server for more information. They can provide insights into how dishes are prepared and may be able to offer suggestions or modifications to accommodate your dietary preferences.

Build Your Own Plate: Many restaurants offer build-your-own options, such as salads, bowls, or wraps, where you can choose your base, toppings, and protein. Take advantage of these customizable options to create a meal that aligns with your flexitarian diet by loading up on vegetables, grains, and plant-based proteins while optionally adding a small portion of meat or other animal products.

Focus on Flavorful Plant-Based Options: Embrace the opportunity to explore and enjoy the diverse world of plant-based cuisine by seeking out dishes that highlight seasonal vegetables, whole grains, and plant-based proteins. Look for flavorful vegetarian or vegan options such as veggie stir-fries, grain bowls, bean-based salads, and plant-based burgers that satisfy your cravings without the need for meat.

Share Small Plates: Consider sharing several small plates or appetizers with your dining companions to sample a variety of flavors and dishes without committing to a large entree. Look for vegetarian or vegan appetizers such as hummus with fresh vegetables, roasted vegetable bruschetta, or crispy tofu bites that offer plenty of flavor and variety.

Be Mindful of Portion Sizes: While dining out, be mindful of portion sizes and avoid overindulging in large portions of meat or other animal products. Instead, aim to fill up on plant-based foods such as vegetables, whole grains, legumes, and nuts, which are often rich in fiber and nutrients and can help you feel satisfied and energized.

By utilizing these strategies, you can navigate dining out as a flexitarian with confidence and enjoyment, savoring delicious and satisfying meals that align with your dietary preferences and values. Remember to be open-minded, flexible, and adventurous in your culinary explorations, and don't hesitate to advocate for your dietary needs and preferences when dining out.

Handling Family Gatherings and Special Events with Grace

Handling family gatherings and special events with grace as a flexitarian involves navigating social situations with confidence, respect, and flexibility. Here are some strategies to help you enjoy these occasions while staying true to your dietary choices:

Communicate Your Dietary Preferences: Before attending family gatherings or special events, communicate your dietary preferences to the host or organizer in a polite and respectful manner. Let them know that you follow a flexitarian diet, which primarily focuses on plant-based foods but occasionally includes meat or other animal products in moderation. Offer to bring a dish to share that aligns with your dietary preferences, ensuring that there will be options available that you can enjoy.

Be Flexible and Adaptable: Understand that not every meal or event will cater perfectly to your dietary choices, and be prepared to be flexible and adaptable in these situations. Focus on finding options that are closest to your dietary preferences while still allowing yourself to indulge occasionally. Look for plant-based dishes or side dishes that you can enjoy, and consider making adjustments or substitutions as needed to accommodate your needs.

Fill Up on Plant-Based Foods: Prioritize filling up on plant-based foods such as fruits, vegetables, whole grains, legumes, nuts, and seeds during family gatherings and special events. These foods are typically abundant and offer a wide range of flavors, textures, and nutrients to keep you feeling satisfied and energized. Load up your plate with colorful salads, roasted vegetables, whole grain dishes, and plant-based proteins to ensure that you're getting plenty of nourishment.

Practice Portion Control: While it's important to enjoy yourself and indulge in special treats during family gatherings and events, practice portion control to avoid overeating. Be mindful of your hunger and fullness cues, and listen to your body's signals to determine when you've had enough. Choose smaller portions of indulgent foods and balance them out with larger portions of healthier, plant-based options to maintain balance and moderation.

Lead by Example: Show your family and friends that following a flexitarian diet is not only delicious and satisfying but also achievable and sustainable. Lead by example by making conscious and mindful food choices, and share your knowledge and experiences with others who may be curious or interested in learning more. Offer to share recipes, cooking tips, and resources to help inspire others to embrace a more plant-centric approach to eating.

Focus on Enjoying the Company: Ultimately, family gatherings and special events are about coming together to celebrate and enjoy each other's company. Instead of fixating solely on the food, focus on the connections and relationships that make these occasions special. Engage in meaningful conversations, participate in activities, and savor the moments spent with loved ones, knowing that the food is just one part of the overall experience.

By approaching family gatherings and special events with grace, flexibility, and mindfulness, you can navigate social situations with confidence and enjoyment while staying true to your flexitarian lifestyle. Remember to communicate your dietary preferences, be flexible and adaptable, prioritize plant-based foods, practice portion control, lead by example, and focus on enjoying the company of loved ones.

CHAPTER 6
OVERCOMING CHALLENGES AND STAYING MOTIVATED

Dealing with Cravings and Temptations

Dealing with cravings and temptations is a common challenge for many individuals, regardless of their dietary preferences. However, as a flexitarian, you may face additional temptations, especially when navigating situations where meat or other animal products are prevalent. Here are some strategies to help you manage cravings and resist temptations effectively:

Identify Triggers: Pay attention to the situations, emotions, or environmental cues that trigger cravings for certain foods. Whether it's stress, boredom, social pressure, or simply seeing and smelling tempting foods, understanding your triggers can help you develop strategies to cope with cravings more effectively.

Plan Ahead: Anticipate situations where you're likely to encounter cravings or temptations and plan ahead to mitigate their impact. For example, if you know you'll be attending a barbecue or family gathering with lots of meat-centric dishes, eat a satisfying and nutritious meal beforehand to help curb your appetite and reduce the likelihood of overindulging.

Keep Healthy Options Handy: Stock your kitchen and pantry with plenty of healthy and satisfying options that align with your flexitarian diet. Having nutritious snacks and ingredients readily available can help you make healthier choices when cravings strike. Fill your fridge with fresh fruits and vegetables, whole grains, nuts, seeds, and plant-based proteins to keep temptation at bay.

Practice Mindful Eating: Slow down and practice mindful eating to become more attuned to your body's hunger and fullness cues. Before reaching for a snack or indulging in a craving, pause and ask yourself whether you're truly hungry or if you're eating out of habit, boredom, or emotion. Choose foods that nourish your body and provide lasting satisfaction rather than fleeting pleasure.

Find Healthy Substitutes: When cravings strike, satisfy them with healthier alternatives that still provide the flavors and textures you crave. For example, if you're craving something salty and crunchy, reach for air-popped popcorn or roasted chickpeas instead of potato chips. If you're craving something sweet, opt for fresh fruit, a small piece of dark chocolate, or a naturally sweetened dessert made with wholesome ingredients.

Practice Moderation: Allow yourself to enjoy your favorite treats and indulgences in moderation, without feeling guilty or deprived.

Adopting a flexible and balanced approach to eating allows you to enjoy a wide variety of foods while still prioritizing nutritious options most of the time. Instead of completely avoiding foods you love, focus on portion control and mindful enjoyment to maintain balance and moderation.

Stay Hydrated: Sometimes, feelings of hunger or cravings can be mistaken for thirst. Stay hydrated throughout the day by drinking plenty of water, herbal tea, or other hydrating beverages. Keeping your body properly hydrated can help reduce cravings and keep your appetite in check.

Practice Self-Compassion: Be kind to yourself and practice self-compassion when dealing with cravings and temptations. Remember that it's normal to experience cravings from time to time, and it doesn't mean you've failed or that you're lacking willpower.

Instead of being hard on yourself, acknowledge your feelings without judgment and refocus on making healthier choices moving forward.

By implementing these strategies, you can effectively manage cravings and resist temptations while staying true to your flexitarian lifestyle. Remember that consistency, mindfulness, and self-compassion are key to maintaining a healthy and balanced approach to eating in the long term.

Troubleshooting Common Obstacles

Embarking on a flexitarian diet journey can be both rewarding and challenging. As with any lifestyle change, it's common to encounter obstacles along the way. Here are some common challenges that flexitarians may face and strategies to overcome them:

Lack of Variety: One challenge for flexitarians is finding a variety of plant-based meals that are both satisfying and delicious. To overcome this obstacle, explore different cuisines, cooking techniques, and ingredients to keep your meals interesting and flavorful. Experiment with new recipes, ingredients, and cooking methods to discover a wide range of plant-based dishes that you enjoy.

Social Pressure: Dining out or attending social gatherings where meat is the focus can be challenging for flexitarians. To navigate these situations, communicate your dietary preferences to friends, family, and restaurant staff in advance. Offer to bring a dish to share that aligns with your flexitarian diet, and focus on filling up on plant-based options while still allowing yourself to enjoy small portions of meat or other animal products if desired.

Convenience: Convenience foods and fast food options often prioritize meat-based dishes, making it challenging for flexitarians to find convenient meal options on the go. To address this challenge, plan and prepare meals in advance whenever possible. Batch cook meals on weekends, stock up on frozen fruits and vegetables, and keep pantry staples like canned beans, grains, and sauces on hand for quick and easy meals during busy weekdays.

Nutritional Balance: Ensuring adequate nutrition on a flexitarian diet requires careful planning to meet your body's needs for essential nutrients. To overcome this obstacle, focus on incorporating a wide variety of plant-based foods into your diet, including fruits, vegetables, whole grains, legumes, nuts, seeds, and plant-based proteins. Consider consulting with a registered dietitian or nutritionist to ensure that you're meeting your nutritional needs and supplementing as needed.

Time Constraints: Balancing work, family, and other responsibilities can make it difficult to prioritize meal planning and preparation. To address this challenge, streamline your meal prep process by batch cooking, meal prepping, and using time-saving kitchen gadgets and appliances. Choose quick and easy recipes that require minimal ingredients and preparation time, and prioritize convenience without sacrificing nutrition.

Budget Constraints: Eating a primarily plant-based diet can be cost-effective, but specialty plant-based products and organic produce can be expensive. To overcome budget constraints, focus on affordable plant-based staples such as beans, lentils, rice, pasta, oats, frozen fruits and vegetables, and bulk grains and legumes. Shop for seasonal produce, buy in bulk, and look for sales and discounts to save money on groceries.

Emotional Eating: Using food as a coping mechanism for stress, boredom, or other emotions can derail your efforts to maintain a healthy flexitarian diet. To address emotional eating, practice mindfulness and self-awareness to identify triggers and develop alternative coping strategies such as exercise, meditation, journaling, or talking to a trusted friend or therapist.

By recognizing and addressing common obstacles, flexitarians can overcome challenges and stay committed to their dietary goals. With patience, persistence, and a positive mindset, you can successfully navigate the ups and downs of a flexitarian lifestyle and enjoy the many benefits of eating a primarily plant-based diet.

Cultivating Long-Term Sustainability in Your Flexitarian Lifestyle

Maintaining a flexitarian lifestyle over the long term requires commitment, planning, and a sustainable approach to eating. Here are some strategies to help you cultivate sustainability and longevity in your flexitarian journey:

Gradual Transition: Instead of making drastic changes overnight, consider gradually transitioning to a flexitarian diet. Start by incorporating more plant-based meals into your diet and gradually reducing your intake of meat and other animal products over time. This gradual approach can help you adjust to new eating habits more easily and sustainably.

Focus on Whole Foods: Emphasize whole, minimally processed foods in your flexitarian diet, including fruits, vegetables, whole grains, legumes, nuts, seeds, and plant-based proteins. These nutrient-dense foods not only provide essential vitamins, minerals, and antioxidants but also support overall health and well-being.

Experiment with Plant-Based Cooking: Get creative in the kitchen and experiment with plant-based cooking techniques, flavors, and ingredients. Explore new recipes, cuisines, and cooking methods to keep your meals exciting and satisfying. Experimenting with plant-based cooking can help you discover new favorite dishes and make the transition to a flexitarian diet more enjoyable and sustainable.

Meal Planning and Preparation: Plan your meals ahead of time and prepare ingredients in advance to streamline your cooking process and save time during busy weekdays. Batch cooking, meal prepping, and using leftovers creatively can help you stay on track with your flexitarian diet even when life gets hectic. Consider creating a weekly meal plan and grocery shopping list to ensure that you have everything you need for nutritious and delicious meals throughout the week.

Listen to Your Body: Pay attention to your body's hunger and fullness cues, as well as how different foods make you feel. Notice how plant-based meals impact your energy levels, digestion, and overall well-being compared to meals that include meat or other animal products. Tuning into your body's signals can help you make informed choices about which foods to include in your flexitarian diet and cultivate a sustainable approach to eating that supports your health and vitality.

Stay Informed: Stay informed about the latest research, trends, and developments in plant-based nutrition and flexitarianism. Keep an open mind and be willing to adapt your dietary choices based on new information and insights. Stay connected with online communities, social media groups, and reputable sources of information to stay inspired, motivated, and informed on your flexitarian journey.

Practice Flexibility and Balance: Embrace flexibility and balance in your flexitarian lifestyle by allowing yourself to enjoy a wide variety of foods and flavors in moderation. There's no one-size-fits-all approach to flexitarianism, so listen to your body, honor your cravings, and find a balance that works for you. Remember that occasional indulgences are part of a healthy and sustainable approach to eating, so don't be too hard on yourself if you deviate from your plan from time to time.

By cultivating long-term sustainability in your flexitarian lifestyle, you can enjoy the many benefits of a primarily plant-based diet while still allowing for flexibility and enjoyment in your eating habits. With patience, perseverance, and a commitment to health and well-being, you can successfully maintain a flexitarian lifestyle for years to come.

CONCLUSION

Embracing Balance and Wellness Through Flexitarianism

In conclusion, flexitarianism offers a balanced and sustainable approach to eating that promotes both personal wellness and environmental sustainability. By primarily focusing on plant-based foods while occasionally incorporating meat or other animal products in moderation, flexitarians can enjoy the benefits of a diverse and nutrient-rich diet while still allowing for flexibility and enjoyment in their eating habits.

Throughout this journey, we've explored the principles of flexitarianism and learned how to navigate common challenges and obstacles. We've discovered the importance of incorporating a variety of plant-based foods into our diet, prioritizing whole, minimally processed ingredients, and practicing mindful eating to stay attuned to our body's needs.

We've also explored strategies for handling social situations, dining out, and managing cravings while staying true to our flexitarian lifestyle. By communicating our dietary preferences effectively, planning and preparing meals in advance, and focusing on nutritious and satisfying options, we can navigate any situation with confidence and grace.

Ultimately, embracing balance and wellness through flexitarianism is about finding what works best for us as individuals. It's about honoring our bodies, our taste preferences, and our values while still enjoying the pleasures of food and eating. It's about making conscious and mindful choices that support our health, the well-being of animals, and the health of the planet.

As we continue on our flexitarian journey, let's remember to approach our dietary choices with curiosity, compassion, and flexibility. Let's celebrate the abundance and diversity of plant-based foods while still allowing ourselves the occasional indulgence. Let's embrace balance and wellness through flexitarianism, knowing that we're making a positive impact on our health, our communities, and the world around us.

Together, we can cultivate a more sustainable and compassionate approach to eating that nourishes our bodies, supports our values, and promotes greater harmony with the natural world. Let's continue to embrace the journey of flexitarianism with open hearts and minds, knowing that every meal we choose is an opportunity to create positive change for ourselves and the planet.

RESOURCES

Additional Reading, Websites, And Tools For Further Support

As you continue your journey toward embracing a flexitarian lifestyle, there are numerous resources available to support and inspire you along the way. Whether you're looking for recipe ideas, nutritional information, or guidance on navigating social situations, these resources can provide valuable insights and practical tips to help you succeed. Here are some recommended resources to explore:

Books:

- **"The Flexitarian Diet:** The Mostly Vegetarian Way to Lose Weight, Be Healthier, Prevent Disease, and Add Years to Your Life" by Dawn Jackson Blatner

- **"The VB6 Cookbook:** More than 350 Recipes for Healthy Vegan Meals All Day and Delicious Flexitarian Dinners at Night" by Mark Bittman
- **"The Plant-Based Solution:** America's Healthy Heart Doc's Plan to Power Your Health" by Joel K. Kahn, MD

Websites and Blogs:

- **The Flexitarian** - A comprehensive website dedicated to flexitarianism, offering recipes, meal plans, articles, and tips for incorporating more plant-based foods into your diet.
- **Forks Over Knives** - A popular website and documentary focused on the benefits of a plant-based diet, offering recipes, meal plans, success stories, and educational resources.
- **Minimalist Baker** - A food blog specializing in simple, plant-based

recipes that are easy to prepare and packed with flavor.

- **NutritionFacts.org** (https://www.nutritionfacts.org/ - A science-based website run by Dr. Michael Greger, offering evidence-based information on the health benefits of a plant-based diet, including videos, articles, and resources.

Apps:

- **HappyCow** - A popular app that helps you find vegan, vegetarian, and veg-friendly restaurants and cafes near you, making it easier to dine out as a flexitarian.

- **MyFitnessPal** - A comprehensive food and nutrition tracking app that can help you monitor your intake of nutrients, calories, and macronutrients, whether you're following a flexitarian diet or any other eating plan.

- **Plant Jammer** - An innovative cooking app that helps you create delicious plant-based meals using ingredients you already have on hand, making it easy to improvise and get creative in the kitchen.

Social Media:

- **Instagram** - Follow hashtags such as #flexitarian, #plantbased, and #meatlessmonday for recipe inspiration, meal ideas, and tips from fellow flexitarians and plant-based enthusiasts.
- **Facebook Groups** - Join online communities and groups dedicated to flexitarianism, vegetarianism, and plant-based living to connect with like-minded individuals, share resources, and seek support and advice.

Podcasts:

- **The Plant-Based Podcast** - Hosted by plant-based nutrition experts, this podcast explores the latest research, trends, and insights in the world of plant-based living.

- **Nutrition Rounds Podcast** - Hosted by Dr. Danielle Belardo, this podcast features interviews with leading experts in plant-based nutrition and lifestyle medicine, offering practical advice and inspiration for improving your health through diet.

By exploring these resources and seeking support from the flexitarian community, you can gain valuable knowledge, inspiration, and encouragement to help you thrive on your flexitarian journey. Whether you're looking for recipe ideas, nutritional information, or guidance on navigating social situations, these resources can empower you to make informed choices and embrace a more balanced and sustainable approach to eating.

9 798888 805776